Giving Care, Taking Care

Support for the Helpers

Sherokee Ilse

ACKNOWLEDGMENTS

I am deeply grateful to the many people who so willingly shared their time, expertise, stories and ideas. Such books as this one are a tribute to the collaboration and sharing nature of many. A special thanks to the following:

Inez Anderson, Associate Manager Perinatal Loss
Janet Bleyl, Executive Director, Triplet Connection
Judith Benkendorf, M.S., Georgetown University
Patricia Evilsizer, R.N., Director Perinatal Loss Program
Kathy Floyd, RTS Bereavement Coordinator
Mary Funk, R.N. Manager Perinatal Loss, Mercy Hospital
Richard B. Gilbert, M.Div., FAAGC, Director Connections-Spiritual Links
Rabbi Earl Grollman, Ph.D.
Suzanne Helzer, R.N.C., C.C.E., RTS Bereavement Coordinator
Joan Klehr, R.N.C., Director of Nursing Services
Catherine Lammert, R.N., Exec. Director, SHARE, Pregnancy & Infant Loss Support, Inc.
Lara Palincsar, M.S.
Michele B. Prince, M.S., C.G.C., Georgetown University Medical Center
Jeri E. Reutenauer, M.S., Genetic Counselor, Georgetown University Medical Center
Fran Rybarik, R.N., M.P.H., Director, RTS Bereavement Services
Rhonda Tomei, M.A., Licensed Professional Counselor

10 9 8 7 6 5 4 3 2 1   96 97 98 Printed in the United States of America
Cover design: Bob Wasiluk and Tim Nelson, deRuyter Nelson Publications
Printing: Lakeland Press   Editor: Carol Frick
Copyright ©1996 by Sherokee Ilse
For additional copies write to:
Wintergreen Press
    3630 Eileen Street
    Maple Plain, MN 55359
    (612) 476-1303

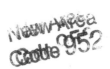

U.S. $10.50

ISBN 1-883525-01-2

CONTENTS

A circle
of unending
love and compassion

Life is a circle—
of giving love
and being loved,
of giving care
and receiving care,
a circle of
unending compassion.

To give is to receive.
As you sow,
so shall you reap.

In giving to others,
you shall receive tenfold.
To give *is* to receive.

Life is a circle,
a circle of unending love.

Sherokee Ilse

We cannot shine if we have not taken time to fill our lamps with oil.
Heartland Sampler

INTRODUCTION

Whether you are a volunteer, a paid professional care provider working with families in crisis, or you are caring for a chronically ill family member, this book is for you. Since little training is given to caregivers on death, dying, bereavement and self-care it seemed appropriate to create a practical resource. *Giving Care, Taking Care* is purposely written not as an academic dissertation, but as a warm gift of concern that will speak to your human, personal side. You may find some sections more relevant to you, some less. Use what touches you and let the rest go for now.

As human beings in the helping professions and family or friends who care for ailing loved ones, we spend much time and energy giving to and nurturing others. We want their journey to be less painful, so we share resources and options, encourage, teach and assist. We hurt when they are in pain and truly care or we wouldn't be doing this work as we give of ourselves and share our gifts.

With every close relationship we form, and with every tragedy we help someone live through, often the rewards are intangible and the price we pay is real. We cannot help but be affected by people's pain. We live it within our hearts. Sharing this experience impacts us, often in pain-filled ways, especially when we cannot take away someone's hurt.

Like you, I have lived, and continue to do so, in both realms. As a hurting soul I have experienced sorrow and tragedy—three babies have died along with my dear mother and grandparents. I have some knowledge of what grieving is like and how important it is to have caring support from professionals and friends who touched me on my journey.

I will never forget meeting our new midwife, Monica, who delivered the bad news that our full term baby had died before birth. She was deeply touched to the point of tears. Her sensitive care and notes over the years further bore that out. She, a perfect stranger, became connected to my husband and me in such special ways. What opened the door was her sensitivity and her willingness to enter our puddle of pain. For this she paid a price; clearly it hurt her to be with us. But I know for certain she also found great satisfaction in helping us through such a difficult time.

As a support person, author and speaker on the subject of bereavement, I have had many opportunities to "be there" for others in pain. This is a far more challenging role than most people outside the caregiving fields realize. The struggles—what to say, how to help, when to call or visit, and the "if only I would haves..."— are endless. The nightly prayers on their behalf and the fears that this too might happen to us or someone we love can be overwhelming at times. The physical and mental strain, along with spiritual questions can take a toll. Often we feel empty and drained, yet our care must continue. People are counting on us.

I have been touched and often overwhelmed with sorrow and pain while supporting others through tragedy, yet the sense of satisfaction has made it personally rewarding. I hope and believe that positives have also come to those I have cared for. I can only hope that my support and compassion has been like warm hugs and small, glowing lights in their long, lonely tunnel of pain.

The needs and the process that both the griever and the helper go through are similar—the feelings, the failings, and the fears. Both also need to keep themselves at the top of the taking care list in order to be there for others. As you travel your own journey and find yourself beside others who are in need of support, may you find balance, satisfaction, comfort and the special gifts that are surely to come. Seek patience with yourself and those who lash out at you in their pain. And may you be able to look back and say that you have been important in the circle of care and compassion.

Knowing that the problems are great as you seek to fulfill your mission to be with people in pain, remember—if you are to give good care to others you must first take care of yourself and understand your appropriate role in guiding and supporting them. That is what this book is about. As Rabbi Earl Grollman states, "If I am not for myself, who is?" If you are to give from your well, it must have water. If you are to shine, your lamp must be filled with oil.

GIVING CARE

There are many aspects involved in giving good care. You may be seeking validation for the level of care you already give and suggestions for improvement. At different times you may feel stimulated and excited, content and satisfied, overwhelmed and inadequate, or even exhausted and worn out. Your challenge is one shared by many—balancing the desire and need to help others while maintaining your physical, emotional and spiritual health. This is vital for yourself, your family, who also need you to be a loving, contributing member, and for those you care for who depend on your well-being.

This book is divided into two parts. This section focuses on the *caregiving* part of the equation—your caregiving style, your role and the benefits and difficulties of helping those in need. The second section is full of strategies and challenges for *taking* care of yourself.

Explore within yourself why you are a caregiver and how it affects you, as well as explore ways to be more effective. Find ways to stretch and grow. Ask yourself the hard questions that need to be asked and remember that this is not a science. There are no clear or *right* answers here. It is a human experiment that continues all through your life. You may grow and learn, but it's likely that you will never feel fully satisfied about each interaction and relationship. This is the nature of humanness and the lack of perfection. However, perfection is not what is really helpful or needed. The most profound and helpful things you can do may be the most simple, if you will allow yourself to risk giving them.

The gift of self

I will work in my own way, according to the light within me.
    —Lydia Maria Child, *You Can't Afford the Luxury of a Negative Thought*

You are special and unique. Your light shines in its own way. As you care for others you have probably already learned that your style is unlike anyone else's. It never seems to work to use another's words or approach exactly. What works best is what comes from your heart and your own experience. While you can learn ideas, techniques and tips from others, they will only be effective if you modify them, to make them your own. Your gifts to others must come from inside you, then they will be honored and appreciated.

Being there is the ultimate gift you can give. It is not necessary to have the exact words or correct actions. Even unhelpful support and words will be forgiven if your attitude of care and concern shines through. What is important is what is in your heart. This is the gift of self!

Everyone has much to share with others if they are willing. You do not have to be a highly trained professional or have years of experience in the field to make a difference in people's lives. A caring smile, gentle words, or even compassion expressed through silence are all things that you can offer to another. These are important and necessary to all humans in crisis; this is what is remembered and appreciated over time. When this humanness and compassion are combined with expertise, families will benefit and so will their care providers. If you work with other professionals also give of yourself to your colleagues, especially to newcomers to the caregiving role. They will benefit from your mentoring during the rough spots of their early days. So take stock of your gifts, your personality and experiences, then combine them with your professional skills and knowledge. Be sure you share them when you sit beside someone who is hurting. ✛List your three greatest strengths you bring to others in need.✛

Supporting people who are grieving

Grieving is as natural as crying when you are hurt, sleeping when you are tired, eating when you are hungry, or sneezing when your nose itches. It is nature's way of healing a broken heart.
　　　　　—Doug Manning, *Don't Take My Grief Away*

Most people are afraid of and will do just about anything to avoid grief. The pain seems too much to bear, especially in our "don't worry, be happy society." It is the antithesis of everything we strive for. Yet, loss and the process that follows happens to everyone (unless they die first). Whether it is the tragedy of death, job loss, health problems, financial problems, marriage and family problems, natural disasters or other trauma, when a change occurs and a dream is lost, there are normal feelings of loss and mourning. These behaviors are an adaptation to the loss.

Grief can be delayed but, most experts agree, it cannot be denied. Therefore, while the fear of living through such sorrow and sadness or anger is natural, it is vital that encouragement and support be given to the victims, as well as the care providers, to face the pain and tackle the journey of mourning the loss. Much is written on this issue, see the Appendix. You may want to expand your knowledge base.

Styles of caregiving

Exploring styles of care is an intriguing exercise. I propose the following categories to contemplate. See if you can relate to any of them. Like most people, you will probably find you have been in each of these roles at some time or another:

Avoiders, sometimes known as the silent types—
"If I don't say anything they will be better off. After all, my words may cause them more pain than they are already feeling," or "I don't know how to help, there is nothing I can do, so why try?" or "If we don't talk about this it will go away," are common reactions offered by the avoider when they come in close contact with people in tragedy. Reviewing medical facts or details is common, rather than acknowledging feelings. They are protecting the victims (as well as themselves) from making mistakes and facing the pain. They genuinely don't know what to say or how to help, so they believe that no words are better than wrong words.

Saviors/Protectors, also known as rescuers—
They are convinced they know what the victim must do in order to feel better and be saved. "Trust me," the savior/protector may say, "I have the experience to know what will work best for someone in this situation."

In their years of professional and personal experience they may feel they have come to know the answers and may freely offer advice

5

on behalf of the one in pain. They seem to be motivated by desperately wanting to "fix it." They want the hurting person to benefit from their experienced counsel and thus be spared the difficult and painful consequences. Savior/protectors usually do this because they genuinely care and believe they have the answers to others' problems. This may seem a worthy goal, but it really is the wrong strategy. The main problem relates to control—they have it, the victim doesn't. This can keep the one in pain weak and vulnerable, feeling low and not trusting their own judgment.

The savior/protectors may be attempting to protect others from a worse tragedy and the resulting sorrow, but it does not stop there. Most likely they are also trying to protect themselves from experiencing this pain. For instance, if they focus on the positive, the future, and what is hopeful they can avoid the feelings of inadequacy and discomfort that come with the pain of the moment.

Advice givers
"It is God's will," "Time heals," "Get used to it (or deal with it)," "Be happy and put it behind you," are the kinds of advice often given by this type of caregiver.

Close cousins to the savior/protectors, the advice givers are offering answers and suggestions to make the situation better. They probably want to help the hurting person "move on." They are full of words of wisdom that are usually shared in a genuine attempt to help. Advice givers share traits with the previous caregiving styles, in that they also feel inadequate about how to *really* help, so they try harder to come up with answers.

Buck-ups
These people believe the best way to recover is, "Get back on the horse," "Don't let this get you down," "Tomorrow is another day." The past is over in the eyes of these people. There is no reason to cry over spilled milk. According to the buck-ups, dwelling on pain only adds to the problem and prevents healing, much like picking at a scab rather than just letting it be.

Buck-ups often have the words of wisdom and the timetable to go with it. They believe their behaviors will help others feel better. They tend to stop talking about the problem(s) within days or weeks in hopes the hurting person will move on and be done.

Puddle sitters

Unlike the buck-ups, the puddle sitters plop themselves in the middle of the puddle of pain and memories to just "be" with the person in pain. They encourage dwelling and wallowing in the misery for awhile, believing that expressing one's feelings is important in the healing process. Rather than viewing "dwelling" and "talking" as picking at a scab, the puddle sitter considers the loss a wound that needs to be drained to rid the body of the toxins.

It seems essential that those in crisis have a few puddle sitters close by. In his book, *Understanding Mourning* Glen Davidson, Ph.D. describes his study of bereavement for the past decade. He shares that having a support network (a contingency of puddle sitters, if you will) is most important to regain health after a significant loss.

Explore your styles of caregiving, your needs, expectations and the real message behind your words. You may find you move from one style to another. When you feel vulnerable or hurt you will give different care than when you are strong and confident. You may experiment with different techniques and styles. As you grow and change, how you care for people will change. ✦Which styles do you use most often? How effective have you been?✦

No matter how you help those who surround you, recognize and remember that you have neither the right nor the ability to take away people's emotional pain. They will heal, recover, find moments of peace or thankfulness on their own timetable and in their own way. Your presence and support as they travel that journey will be immensely helpful. Give of your heart and care enough to be with them; this is a profound gift.

The fact that you also feel pain as a professional or as the care provider is understandable; it comes with the territory. Do not try to deny your own pain or seek magical, speedy cures, but rather allow yourself to grieve and work toward healing in your own way. This attitude will help you and those you support.

7

Your role in helping deal with grief and loss

Grief is not an enemy—it is a friend. It is the natural process of walking through hurt and growing because of the walk. Let it happen. Stand up tall to friends and to yourself and say, 'Don't take my grief away from me. I deserve it, and I am going to have it. —Doug Manning, *Don't Take My Grief Away*

It is uncomfortable to care for people experiencing emotional pain. You may feel your goal, your very job, is to relieve them of their pain, to make them better. This is true in the physical sense, especially if you are connected to the medical community. But when it comes to emotions and faith, the purpose of healing and support is not to remove the pain, but to live through it and with it. Eventually the physical pain may be lessened, but the pain of the soul and the emotions are not so easily diminished. No amount of wishful thinking, thankfulness for what they do have, or looking forward rather than backward, will erase the pain. The only way out of this tunnel of sorrow is *through*, facing bit by bit the cause of the pain and the reactions from the loss, before the healing and building of new dreams can come.

A common response when someone is crying uncontrollably or is expressing sadness, anger or fear is the desire to lessen or take away their grief. Avoiding painful subjects and steering their attention from their pain may seem like a help, but in fact it does the opposite. It weakens their own natural coping techniques.

No human being has the right or responsibility to emotionally heal someone else. Don't try to shorten another's tunnel of grief. It is common to worry too much about saying the right thing and to attempt to keep the the hurting person from crying or showing too much anger. Rather than this, your attempts at comfort can affirm and validate, helping them understand that *having the pain and experiencing the loss is okay and necessary in order to feel better.* After all, their loved one, or their dream, is worth crying over and worth missing. This is a high tribute to who or what has been lost. Their lives can no longer go on the same. What has been lost is usually a treasure, not a trinket to be missed for but a short time.

Why not begin (or continue) the relationship knowing that it is not your place to try to make it better? Rather, share your compassion and sit in their puddle, where they may need to wallow, complain, wail, cry, and show anger. This relieves you of the pressure of trying to make someone better and allows you to be your kind, caring self. You can be more free to look in their eyes and reach out to their hearts without an agenda. It's helpful to sit down beside them, not across,which can be interpreted as talking at them. Share silence, your presence, hugs, or a hand on their arm. Don't try to fix it. Listen and don't judge. Express your concern and your own feelings. Teach them about grief and their options. You may be able to help them find calm or short-term moments of peace. Be careful not to take over; families need to find the answers themselves. Yet, they need you to be there and to know that you care.

You are also affected in ways you may not always realize or want to admit as you care for others. You may be reminded of your own sorrows and troubles, and in trying to protect families from too much sadness, you may also be protecting yourself. This is normal, yet not helpful to either of you in the long run. This can hinder giving good, objective care.

Rescuer or helper?

I think we need to realize our job does not include removing or curing someone's pain. This is so important. There are limits to what we can do, but what we do does make such a difference. Each of us has something to answer and something to give.
—Mary Funk, R.N.

To delve into your role further lets explore two types of caregiving:

Rescuer: One who takes charge and control of another who is vulnerable and in need of help, a protector—
The responsibility and decision making are usually controlled by the rescuer; therefore, the results, the credit and the blame can be believed to be attributed to the rescuer. Being needed and making a difference can feel good when a life is saved. But when things don't go well, the person being cared for isn't healing, or the decisions made turn out to be poor ones with terrible consequences, the rescuer is the first to be blamed.

Many care providers fall into the trap of trying too hard to help others, especially when they sense that the victim wants to be rescued. Caregivers may attempt to be the hero, by trying to take away the victim's emotional pain. This type of helping can become inappropriate and excessive. The rescuer may not realize this hurts more than help.

Playing the rescuer is a dangerous role. It involves boundary issues. The rescued one gets the message that their caregiver knows best and will take care of them. They stay needy and dependent, feeling weak with a lowered self-esteem. They can quickly come to rely on the rescuer. Dependency sometimes leads to mutual resentment.

One could ask, is the rescuer helping others for the sake of helping them, or so their own needs might be met? The good feelings that come from making a significant difference in someone's life can be intoxicating and motivating. With that much power and control, this type of caregiving is easily perpetuated. But, when things go wrong, or the vulnerable individual has more problems, the rescuer is often the first to be blamed.

I realize now that I had confused who the real benefactor was as I tried to help everyone with the problems they brought to my doorstep. I kept telling myself they needed me, when in fact, I needed to be needed and seen as a helping, all-wise person.
—Sue Vineyard

Helper: One who assists, stands by and supports another in a non judgmental fashion, an advocate or facilitator—
A helper does *not* take charge, but is available, with resources and support, to listen, share, and offer information, but not solve the problem for the hurting individual. When things go badly the helper is not to be blamed or credited, but rather thanked for standing by in tough times.

This is a much healthier position to be in. It is clear that the person in our care is the decision maker and ultimately in control of their own life. The helper is there to assist, guide, teach, share options, talk about the short- and long-term issues, while acknowledging that it is up to the family members. Of course, if there are emergency decisions to make or immediate action is needed to ease the crisis, the helper may wish to take charge temporarily, relinquishing that role as soon as possible.

It is critical that you recognize the distinct difference between these two roles. One gives you responsibility (and control) to make it better and do the right thing and the other gives the control to the vulnerable person.

Wherever possible shift the power and responsibility back to the individual or family. You may need to teach them about their options and rights. Guide them in their decision making so it is not done in a narrow context with the focus only on today.

Examine your role and clarify your boundaries, then respect them. Release yourself from the pressure to do and say the "right" things. Let down some of your defenses and be open to the moment and the needs of the person in your care. ✠Review times you have acted as a rescuer and a helper. How were the situations and results alike and different?✠

Searching for answers as a way of comforting

He's brain dead. The words struck like a torch searing through me just below my sternum. What did I do wrong? Why did this tragedy happen? Could I have overlooked something?...I am angry but I don't know where to direct the anger except internally. How can I explain this tragedy to his parents and try to comfort them? Who is going to comfort me? All the methods and words I have learned, over the past 20 plus years of practicing pediatrics, to use to give solace and comfort to grieving parents at this moment sound like rationalizations...I am still looking for answers. Perhaps life is like something Gertrude Stein once said, 'There ain't no answer. There ain't going to be any answer. There never has been an answer. That's the answer.' —Dr. Alvin Freund

It is common for caregivers to attempt to offer families answers or reasons, for medical, emotional or spiritual challenges. You may fill in silent or painful moments with words, advice and your view about what has happened and why. The hurting person may lead you to believe that they too are looking for answers. Sometimes the need for answers becomes a way to hide from the pain and facing the grief. It can also cloud the real fears and questions. Be careful

11

that you don't use either the search or the inability to find answers in ways that don't help you or others. ⊕Think of times you have sought answers that were beyond the needs of the hurting person. What could you do instead?⊕

Am I doing enough? Sometimes I feel guilty and inadequate.

If you ever ask yourself this or wonder if you are going about this in the "right" way, you can feel secure that you are not alone. This is something everyone feels, often on a daily basis. You may feel guilty and inadequate that there is not more that you can do. You may look enviously at how others behave, give care and handle the daily pressures. It is because you *do care* and maybe because you wish to be the perfect care provider that the feelings of inadequacy surface. You cannot adopt someone else's style, methods or techniques and still be yourself. Appreciate what you do well and be glad for those gifts you are able to share, then build upon them as you continue to grow.

Step back and take a fresh look. Admit that you can't do it all, that you get tired, that you don't always say the right words, don't have the answers and have your own needs on a daily basis. Do what you can to gain perspective.

It will only be in hindsight that you can evaluate how you did, but then your answers will only fit for your care of *that* person, *that* family. You can learn as you go and you can improve over time and with experience. However, admit to yourself that you can never be perfect. You will always have regrets and wonder if you should have done something differently. Learn to live with these feelings, accept them for what they are, strive to use what you have learned next time, and then say to yourself, "I am human. I did the best I could at the time. Tomorrow is a new day and I will take what I have learned and also do my best in the future." Now live and let go.

Can this happen to me?

It is natural to feel vulnerable when you see someone hurting or dying. You may feel that if it can happen to them, it can happen to you and others you love. While you don't want these feelings to interfere with the care you give, you may find them cropping up at times. You may go home and give your children or partner an extra hug. At times you may look around and realize the many things you have in your life to be thankful for. Good health may not be something you can take for granted for awhile. You are reminded again of the vulnerabilities of life and this can be frightening. The feelings you have are ones those in pain can relate to. They too feel vulnerable, as if their invincible bubble has been burst. This common bond may help you understand each other.

If it is your loved one who is ill, it *is* happening to you. You may question how and why this has happened. In the beginning the shock may insulate you to a degree while you go through the motions. After awhile the strain will show, tempers and patience wear down, and fears and worries can overwhelm. What you thought could never happen to you has!

I find it very difficult to ask for help

In your current caregiving role you are often perceived as the "strong one." It may not seem right to ask for help for yourself or to receive support or assistance from others. After all, you must hold it together on behalf of others. You may feel that if you seek support or accept advice you are admitting you can't handle it or will be seen as "weak" or even a "failure." You may feel that you should be able to handle this on your own. However, this is often not realistic. You are not superhuman. Deep down everyone needs support and the help of others.

As a professional, depending on training and experience, you may feel that the pressure to perform appropriately is intense. In the past, care providers were taught to keep their feelings and emotions outside the room of the vulnerable one. The current philosophy tends to encourage care providers to show their humanness and to integrate their personal experiences and feelings with their professional skills in a way that respects self-disclosure issues. One must maintain an appropriate balance. No one expects those in crisis to have to care for the caregiver who has lost focus. You need to maintain your professionalism while sharing some of your feelings and needs—a difficult balance.

13

Many new and young care providers seem to struggle with this issue of showing feelings and admitting they too need help. It's natural to be afraid of making a mistake, saying the wrong thing or being judged as not competent. People look to you to be the strong one, while at the same time wanting sensitive, personalized care. If anything, you will gain more respect and trust from the people you assist when you show your compassion. It's obvious you care and that you are touched. It can show that you are more like them than different from them, which can help you to relate to one another. Seek out senior colleagues for mentoring opportunities as you need assistance during difficult situations.

After writing the previous paragraph and sharing it with many seasoned professionals, I was reminded by most of them, that this also happens to those who have been in the caregiving business for a long time. It's easy to believe that by now they "should" be able to handle all the pain and tragedy; after all, they are experienced and are the role models for their newer colleagues. Their internal message might be, "I know how to keep a distance and maintain my professionalism, therefore I must." In addition, the number of difficult situations and hurting families adds up.

We don't always have to 'be strong' to be strong. Sometimes our strength is expressed in being vulnerable. We even need to fall apart to regroup and stay on track. —Melody Beattie, *The Language of Letting Go.*

Talk with colleagues, seek out counselors, read literature that might aid you. Take your own advice, which you probably readily give to others. Don't try to do this alone; ask for help when you first feel the need. Don't wait until you are hitting the bottom. Practice patience and if need be take a step back from emotional battles or especially painful situations do so. See the second part of this book for more suggestions for staying healthy and strong.

As a lay care provider you are operating out of desire and need, yet may have limited professional skills and few colleagues and friends who are in the same boat to call upon when you need help. Remember, if you wish to remain strong and to be there for your loved one, support and help are necessary for you at many points in this journey.

Whether professional or a lay support person, consider your feelings and vulnerability a special gift of your humanness. It is a vital key in your personal and professional journey, a way to be authentic and honest with yourself and others. Own it and deal with it. Work on keeping things in perspective and using your own resources to support and empower you. Others will probably respect you more for it than if you had continued to act like you are totally self-reliant and need no help from anyone. ⊕What do you do when you feel in over your head? List your support resources. ⊕

It's hard to have empathy if I feel they played a part in causing this tragedy

There are many times when caregivers can look at someone and feel they played an active part in their own disease or tragedy. Drugs, drinking or smoking may have played a role. Maybe they used bad judgment or did other unhealthy things.

It is understandable if you are angry or find it hard to give your genuine empathy to people who you feel put themselves in this position. Admit your feelings to yourself, then find ways to deal with them, preferably outside of earshot from the vulnerable person. If you need to scream it out, write it down, or share it with someone else (be careful that it is not a relative or friend who may feel hurt by your revelations), do that. Then remind yourself what your commitment is to this person.

Rarely do you know for certain what causes an illness or tragedy, though there certainly are times when it is seems obvious. Whatever the case, judgment and blame are not going to be helpful to this person and their family now. Put yourself in their place—even if you did do something stupid or wrong, if you broke a bone, had a cold or were faced with a serious tragedy as a result, what would you really need? You could beat up on yourself for a long time. Would you need your caregivers to add ammunition to the already volatile situation? If you are honest with yourself, you will probably answer that people need non judgmental tender care, rest and support. No matter how they got there, that part is over. What they have now are the problems and needs of today, this moment. You may need to do some work to deal with your feelings, but can you get beyond it and give the care that is needed? If you, as the caregiver, cannot find it in your heart to give that tender and compassionate care talk with others, your colleagues, supervisor, or other relatives and friends if you are not a professional in this situation. Ask for help from someone else so you can get the space you need to reevaluate your feelings and the hurting person gets the care they need.

Utilizing resources and making referrals

In order to give the best care you can it is imperative that you have identified appropriate resources—the family's and the community's. Resource persons, groups, individuals and helpful written information multiply the aspects of care that can be offered and can relieve the load on you, the caregiver. Who are the people in the family who can help with day-to-day care, offer emotional and, if necessary, financial support? What literature, organizations, support groups and individuals might be of help? In many cases, much of this information is already known and might be collected. Use your skills, supportive friends and colleagues to help gather this information. Then pass it along to the person in need both in written and verbal form at times when they are able to really hear.

When you have reached your limit or feel you have done all you physically and emotionally can it is time to make referrals to others. Ask for help. Be honest with what you can realistically do. Then let go. Where appropriate keep checking in to follow-up what progress is being made and how they are doing.

In summary, the following suggestions may be helpful reminders:

Suggestions to aid in giving good care

- Respect and appreciate the patient/client/person in pain as a unique and loved individual.
- While in their presence, don't talk about them to others.
- Call them by name and if their loved one has died say that person's name out loud.
- Offer specific suggestions of help, rather than the generic "Let me know what I can do." Often, people can't ask for help or don't know exactly what they need.
- Share your heart and your genuine concern, rather than seeking nonexistent magical answers to relieve pain.
- Admit you are not perfect, you are still learning and then let go of the *shoulds* and *musts*.
- During and after the moments of crisis, speak slowly and calmly.
- Watch for messages that they have had enough and are no longer listening (e.g., closed or roving eyes, tight or fidgety body language, or changing the subject). Then take a break.
- Ask questions, share options, teach about short- and long-term consequences, then when possible, give the control back to them.
- Be aware of your own feelings, challenges and grief responses. Work at not projecting your needs and feelings on them.
- Know your boundaries; communicate them. Be a good role model.
- Keep communication channels open and flowing. Ask many questions, including, "What do you understand will happen now?" or "Tell me, what has the doctor or other caregiver told you?"
- Be positive and reaffirming as much as possible. Share hope and give encouragement. However, be careful that you are not overly optimistic or upbeat if the occasion does not warrant it.
- Share realism and honesty.
- Express some of your feelings, talk about the tension and the fears.
- Be honest with yourself about your actual role in helping. Only take on what you really have the skills and *right* to do.
- Instead of *protecting* (protecting often turns into overprotecting, which further complicates the original problem), offer support, guidance and facilitation as they live the journey themselves.
- Don't make promises you can't keep and keep all promises you make.
- Prepare them for what is about to happen and answer questions truthfully, though listen carefully to what is being asked. Sometimes people are only ready to hear part of the answer.
- When in doubt, rather than deciding for them, *check it out*.
- *Be good to yourself; take good care of yourself.*

TAKING CARE

Love yourself and treat yourself well. You deserve it and will be better able to give good care since you have taken good care.
— Anonymous

One of the best gifts to others is taking good care of yourself. As a caregiver you need to put your own oxygen mask on first. Don't get caught in the trap of breathing in toxic fumes while trying to help others—you won't last very long.

Whether you are fairly good at taking care of yourself, need reminders and encouragement, or feel you have a long way to go, read on, seeking ways to challenge yourself. There are no precise answers or strategies for the best way to take good care. Open your mind and heart to seek attitudes and methods that could help you. Then share them with your co-workers, relatives, friends and model them for the people in your care.

The circle of giving comes back to you

Giving is the secret of a healthy life...not necessarily money, but whatever a man has of encouragement and sympathy and understanding.
— John D. Rockefeller, Jr.

The satisfaction and good feelings you have when you support and help someone who needs you cannot be described. The job may be hard, and you are touched by the physical and emotional pain of what the family or patient is going through—but the smile of thanks, the genuine acceptance of help and the appreciation you receive can make all of it worthwhile. This is the "meat" of life, the true meaning of being human and really caring for another. To really touch someone during a crisis in their life is an amazing responsibility and gift. You influence their memories forever.

During those times when you are feeling especially drained or blue, focus on the gifts you have shared with others, and they with you. Remind yourself of the satisfaction you have felt and recognize that you are making a meaningful difference in someone's life. Use that to balance the down and difficult times. If you get letters, cards or phone calls of thanks from people, keep them around on your desk and in your head. Create a "smile file" to read on bad days; make copies for your boss and your employee file. It is okay to "need" this now and again. It keeps us human and humble. It can help you find meaning and satisfaction in the role you are playing in someone's journey.

If you do not work with people on a long-term basis, but rather only see them in the crisis and the short-term following the problems, you miss something very important. Understanding the difference you made in their lives and having an awareness of what helped them and what did not, can give you satisfaction and important information. This helps with closure, making the circle more complete.

You may share the belief that what goes around comes around. Good things will return to you in many ways over your lifetime. Trust and remember that. ⊕List two gifts you have you received from others.⊕

Relationships and support at home and work

I had come to believe at an early age that the most important thing on which we could spend our energy was relationships.
    —Sue Vineyard, *How to Take Care of You So You Can Take Care of Others.*

Keeping solid, supportive relationships is a key to surviving life's difficulties. Studies show that when someone is mourning a loss, the most important factor in regaining health is "a nurturing support network." This same philosophy fits for you in your personal and professional life.

Build a supportive work environment. If you give care in your professional life, support from your co-workers and supervisor is very important in order for if you are to continue to do your job well. Sometimes the politics and the personalities actually add to the stress you and others may feel. You cannot ignore this for very long, yet there may be much that you have no power, or right, to change.

If there is little or no support among your colleagues, you may want to be the one to begin to change that. Be patient, it won't happen in a day or a month, but be persistent. Seek support from one or two others and start small. Find out if others have similar feelings of frustration. Ask how they handle things. Share ideas, feelings and coping techniques. Seek out the people and policies that you feel you may be able to have a positive influence over. Don't go about suggesting change in a negative or threatening way, but rather in an optimistic and positive-based manner. If you really want to enhance your environment, the best place to start is with yourself. When you change your manner of handling things or interact with someone differently you will likely experience things differently. Others may also make changes, but there are no guarantees. Keep in mind that the only one you have control over is *you*.

Many caregivers take time to work out a support system with their peers. In one of my workshops I met NICU nurses who would call in the chaplain to do a service for "their" babies whenever they were feeling really stressed and overwhelmed by the deaths of babies in the nursery. They got together to remember, cry, smile over the good memories and say goodbye. Making time to do this helped them recharge their batteries and be ready to care for the next round of babies and families. Some care providers set up either formal or informal support groups for themselves in their institution or in their community. You don't need an official group to do this, but if a group would help, form one.

When you personally have had a long-term relationship with someone who is dying, or have a loved one who is in crisis you can identify with the struggles of those in your care. It hits home and hurts you. Maybe you are faced with continual losses if you are a funeral director, a hospice volunteer, a clergyperson, or an ICU or NICU nurse. When one loss piles on top of another it can be overwhelming, draining your well of energy and resources. You may feel depleted or empty at times. A key to recharging your batteries is getting that encouragement and understanding you need from a support system.

Whether you are a lay or a professional care provider, support at home and in your community is vital. This is where you can have your faith renewed and your energy revived. Rely on your family, good friends, local resources and faith community to help you when you need it. Chances are others have come to you before; now it is your turn. Think of it as taking turns, giving and receiving. Both are necessary in a relationship. Have some fun, enjoy the people who are dear to you and, when possible, leave your worries and work out of your living room. Of course, there are exceptions to this. Maybe you occasionally seek out a listening ear among your family members. Continue to do so if this is working. Just be careful that you don't burn them out by unloading too much or asking too often. ✛Write out the names of these special people in your life.✛

As you look toward the future, spend more time nurturing relationships—build new ones with people you respect and feel in harmony with, and strengthen ones that maybe you haven't given attention to lately. These people are the ones with whom we can be totally open, honest and vulnerable. We can celebrate with them and share problems with them without feelings of competition or feeling threatened.

Live for today and embrace life

Yesterday is history, tomorrow is a mystery, today is a gift—that's why it's called the present. Appreciate each day to the fullest, enjoy life and laugh about it. —Steve Wilson, M.A.

The troubles and worries of tomorrow can get in our way of living for today. While it is easier said than done, make efforts to experience and enjoy today's sunrise, the flowers or scenery, the kindnesses of others and the family or friends you hold dear. This may help you keep life in perspective and not become too serious or overburdened with what happened yesterday, which cannot be changed, and what may or may not happen tomorrow.

In his book, *Living, Loving & Learning*, Leo Buscaglia writes, " I don't know about you but I don't think what is essential about me is my house or my car or my clothes. What is essential about me? Well, I think what is essential is that I live and *embrace life right now*, wherever I am. I grab it in my arms! Don't spend time crying about yesterday—yesterday is over with! I forgive the past.

I forgive the people who have hurt me. I don't want to spend the rest of my life blaming and pointing a finger. Take yourself in your arms and hug yourself, you sweet old thing! Sure you've screwed up, and sometimes you do dumb things and you forget that you are a human being, but the most wonderful thing about you is that, no matter where you are, you have potential to grow. You are just starting."

It is normal and understandable to get caught up in what we should have or could have done, or what we might do tomorrow. But these worries and guilt feelings can be great distractions from the heart of life and what really matters—our lives, our families, health, relationships and other issues that are happening today. Keep things in perspective, don't become overwhelmed and try not to let problems weigh you down too much. Try to take life less seriously, even if only for moments or hours each day. Live today to the fullest!

If you are feeling overwhelmed and devoid of humor, you may need ideas on how to lighten your life. Below are some simple suggestions meant to encourage you to stretch yourself in as many ways as possible as you work to add lightness to your day.

• Find one comic strip or cartoon in the paper that brings forth a smile or laugh. Share it with someone.
• Look around your home, your environment, your job site and find one simple thing to be thankful for—a sunset, a flower garden, a child, the security of your home, a supportive or kind friend/co-worker, your health or other blessings.
• Learn a joke (from a child if need be, they are usually great at jokes) and tell it to someone. If you are not good at jokes (I can relate to this problem!) practice it a few times. If you blow it, enjoy the moment and make that the joke.
• Examine some of the things that make you feel "crazy" in your environment. Change your view of something, seeking the absurdity or silliness of it.
• Don't watch heavy TV or video dramas on difficult days. Instead rent a comedy, maybe even an old *Three Stooges, Laurel and Hardy* or even *I Love Lucy*.

Facing your own losses

Just as you counsel others to face their feelings and losses, it is important that you do the same. Because you are a care provider, you are not immune from the pain and the need to grieve your losses. In fact, you may be more at risk since your position presents you with many more losses on a weekly basis than most families face at one time. Do you feel vulnerable, tired or overwhelmed? Are you reminded of other painful crises in your life? Does working with this person/family touch your heart with sadness? How do you and your family usually handle pain and loss? Does that method work for you now? Be careful you do not rely on alcohol or other mood altering substances. Caregivers can tend to isolate themselves and turn to their own private pain relievers and therapy.

Whether the losses are old ones revisited or new losses, they are real, they are inside you and they need to be dealt with. The internal emotional pain needs creative expression so it can be released and dispersed. There are many ways to accomplish this process, among them are: talking with friends, family and colleagues, attending support groups, exercise, writing, needlework, music, carving or reaching out to others in a similar situation. You have the same kinds of needs; you must find the coping styles that work for you in your grieving and healing process. Every effort should be made to keep the intense part of your pain from interfering with the care you give. Yet, the pain you feel can be a bond between you and those experiencing trauma. You will need to strike a careful balance.

• Explore your feelings concerning your own personal losses and the losses you face at work.
• Identify those losses you are still struggling to overcome.
• Identify resources that can help you deal with loss.
• Think about your idea of life after death.
• Recognize your personal limitations.
• Actively deal with the patient's death or losses.
• Reduce your own tension by practicing a positive attitude, exercising, and relaxing.

(adapted from) Pediatric Nursing, Jan.-Feb. 1991, *Saying Goodbye in the Intensive Care Unit: Helping Caregivers Grieve.*

Attending memorial and funeral services for people you have cared for can be doubly helpful to the family and to you. You offer them support, showing your genuine concern, and you can be a mourner yourself. The stories told, the memories of how this person lived and died are important. This can be a healthy ritual and time for you, though it won't be easy. But don't pressure yourself to go it feels like too much. ⊕ List three or four losses you have experienced. How did you cope—what and who helped? ⊕

Crying

As you may know crying is a natural response for many people, though not all, that literally releases tension and toxins. This healthful reaction gets mixed reviews in most circles. Its value is usually understood, but the pressure to keep from crying is great. There are some places where it is acceptable—in the sporting arena, at sad movies, and in the shower where no one need know. Give yourself, and the people you care for permission to cry. Express your sadness, frustration, and even anger through crying and other methods that don't hurt anyone. Once you allow crying to be a coping tool you may find that it comes easier and is less embarrassing and upsetting. Be a role model for children and the people in crisis.

Stress, illness and attitude

It's often said that stress is one of the most destructive elements in people's daily lives, but that's only a half truth. The way we react to stress appears to be more important than the stress itself.
—Bernie S. Siegel

Identify and become aware of the stress you are living. How you handle the pressure in your life is important. As you may already know the immune system is depressed immediately after crisis, thus you become more vulnerable to sickness. Dr. Bernie Siegel reports that people who are happy, have a good outlook on life and who find ways to express their feelings are less likely to get cancer and be sick. Conversely, people who are depressed or full of despair, those who have a negative outlook on life, or who keep everything inside and deny problems reduce their immune system and have a higher incidence of illness.

Your attitude makes all the difference in the world. Attitude and its effect on healing has been studied for a long time. Think about how your own attitude affects your life. Do you let things (big and little) get you down and overwhelm you? Do you take the upbeat positive approach when at all possible? When you feel down and depressed, what is your view of your work, family, your self-esteem and the problems you face? Chances are this is also the time when you get sick or don't have the stamina to take on difficult and draining tasks. On the other hand, when you are looking at the sunny side of life, it often takes a lot to darken your sky.

There are specific characteristics among healthy executives in high stress jobs, according to Suzanne Kobasa, a health researcher at the University of Chicago, in *From Burnout to Balance* by Dennis Jaffee and Denise Scott. The specific characteristics she noted include:

• A feeling of control over things that mattered to them
• A greater feeling of involvement in what they were doing
• A desire to seek challenges, take risks and look for a new slant

These executives felt self-reliant, confident and creative. There was a sense of positive personal power. ✛Do you feel control over what's important in your life? List one or two of the challenges you currently face and what you feel you do have control over.✛

People with a positive outlook on life may appear to have smaller problems and less pain. They probably get ill less often, too. Yet, it is not what has happened to them or the degree of their agony, but rather the way in which they view their problems. In the end it is what they do about it that seems to make the difference. You, too, can follow this direction, if you examine and occasionally alter your attitude.

The coping techniques you utilize also make a big difference in your life. There are things you can do to seek good health when feeling overwhelmed or over stressed. These will be continue to be explored later in the book, among them: seeking support and help, eating well and getting plenty of exercise and rest, and finding ways to move the internal pressure and feelings of pain to the outside. You can expand your coping techniques by learning from others. Read the literature and popular press to stretch yourself. Then experiment as you deal with your feelings and needs. ✛List three to five things you do to to deal with your stress. Now list three to five more that you'd like to learn to do or wish you did better.✛

It is never too late to change—if that is what you wish to do.

Leaving your work at the office

Too many times I would leave the office with a headache, thinking of all the things I didn't get done and still had left to do. I suddenly realized that was self-defeating. Now when I close the door I try to take stock of all the things accomplished during the day, including all those crises and jobs that weren't on my list but had to be handled. —Judith Benkendorf, M.S.

At times you may often feel overwhelmed at work and home. Many people today find there is too much to do in too little time with too few people to help. The pressure becomes even more intense when you combine this with working with vulnerable people in pain.

If in your job you continually see people in the acute and early phases of their pain, day in and day out, you miss the opportunity to see them grow and change, moving on with life as they integrate their experience. Look at the whole picture and realize that your work and care *are* helpful. This may aid in your sleeping at night and feeling better about your role in their journey. A card, booklet, a brief phone call or note can be a bright spot in the day for both parties.

When you lack closure, have loose ends, or have little time for completion or follow-up you can be left with an over-all feeling of incompleteness. Find the loose ends or problems that usually bother you after you leave work. Discuss them with others and determine if you can handle them in a better way. You need to make time for closure and debriefing. Then make it a priority to do more to separate your work from your home life. All will benefit if you do this.

I sometimes feel as if I have no more left to give.

"Why can't I get hold of myself?" Your physical and emotional resources are stretched to the limit . You feel like you are losing control. You feel helpless and disorganized. "If only I could run away, anywhere." You need time to collect yourself.
—Rabbi Earl Grollman, *Caring and Coping When Your Loved One is Seriously Ill*

This happens. And it is an important sign to notice, especially if you wish to avoid burnout. You may need some attention, rejuvenation, a temporary fix, or possibly a reevaluation of where you are and what you are doing. It is time to assess yourself. Maybe you are overworked, have excess tension in your life, or your caregiving well needs to be replenished. Take a look at the possible issues you are facing. Does it seem things are out of balance? Is life spinning out of control? ✛On paper make a list of current stressors—who needs you, what problems do you face, what else is going on in your life? Then write down what you are doing to add energy and health into your life. ✛

If you wish to regain strength and energy you will probably need to take the initiative to make some changes. Maybe you could pull back from some of the extra things you are doing and put yourself nearer the top of the list by taking better care of yourself especially now, even if you don't think you have time. By doing that you will likely find more energy, which in turn will help you have a better perspective and work more efficiently.

Make time for quiet contemplation and introspection, a chance to drift and think or not think. Talk with others—clergy, a counselor or a good, reliable friend. Look within and without as you remind yourself of the importance of taking care of yourself. Determine whether you need to do more for yourself while continuing this work, or you need a vacation or a longer break. Now is the time to do something about these feelings, before you get sick, harm those in your care more than help, or dig yourself into a dark hole. You are not the first to feel this way, but what you do at this juncture is critical.

Could it be burnout I am feeling?

How do you know if this truly is burnout or if you are just in a temporary low mood and need some attention or a break? Some signs of burnout, or even depression, might include:

- A callousness or reserve that wasn't there before, and seems to be getting in the way of offering people the sensitivity and support they need
- Feeling overly sad and depressed often to the degree that you have trouble making decisions or doing your job
- Able to give less care and concern to family, friends, clients or patients than is expected of you, yet you don't seem to mind
- Excessive anger and bitterness toward your job and/or the people in your care
- Severely decreased feelings of empathy or compassion for those who are in need of your care
- Using alcohol or other mood altering drugs excessively to cope and make it through the day or evening
- Spending more time complaining about the families you serve and your job than noticing what is going well and what you like
- Feeling stuck, out of control and helpless

These might be some of the signs that your attitude is in serious trouble. You may have gone beyond fatigue and typical stress and instead have lost much of your compassionate heart. Yes, this could be burnout or possibly even depression. If you have many of the above feelings or if you wonder why you are in this profession (or doing this work) and worry whether you will survive the next few weeks/months, it is time to look at your current situation seriously. ✛If you think you might be facing depression or burnout commit to talk with someone and seek help as soon as possible.✛

Talk with a respected support person, your supervisor, the human relations department, a counselor or clergyperson about what you can do to gain back perspective and a positive attitude. It takes much work to renew yourself. Taking a vacation or a break may be a good start, but may not be enough. Often burnout is accelerated by poor physical health and inadequate self-care.

Attitude plays a critical role; it is the one thing you can control, with work and help. If you want to make appropriate changes you will and can. It is up to you; all change begins with you. Your attitude and decisions to handle something, quit something, get extra training, seek additional support, or take care of your physical, emotional and spiritual needs will make the difference. You might want to ask yourself why it is that caregivers are so good at strongly recommending healthy behaviors, but ignoring it for themselves?

In the meantime be patient with yourself and seek patience with those in your care. Do things to calm yourself such as take deep breaths, leave any volatile situation for awhile or take a "mental" walk. Recognize when you are not able to help someone because you have had enough, are overwhelmed or have lost patience.

Exercise and nutrition

The importance of exercise, good nutrition and taking vitamins should not be undervalued. There are many physical and psychological benefits. They include feeling more alert, having a better attitude about life and yourself and a better ability to manage stress.

Physical fitness consists of many components and there are a number of ways to become physically fit. You need not exercise strenuously to gain fitness. Regularity is important, however. Exercising three to five times a week is a good goal. Both aerobic and muscle toning workouts can be done.

The benefits of vigorous exercise are to improve the functioning of the lungs and circulatory system, delay the degenerative changes of aging, increase ability to transport oxygen throughout your body and strengthen the heart. During exercise endorphins are released and produce a relaxed and often euphoric state. Recent studies have found that exercise lifts the spirits of even clinically depressed individuals.

If you have not exercised regularly, are overweight, have symptoms of a disease or have other risk factors, you should consult a physician before you begin an exercise program.

Eating regular and well-balanced meals is important for a sound mind and body. The current thinking suggests that eating a diet of fresh fruit and vegetables combined with high carbohydrates and low fat will provide good nutrition for you. You may notice mood swings, anxiety or short temper when you miss meals. It is often advised to eat small meals throughout the day rather than saving up for one big meal. Probably the worst time to eat a big meal is in the evening. This may actually keep you awake at the very time when you seek calm, rest and sleep. When this is combined with daily exercise, you will feel better emotionally and physically.

If you are feeling depressed, full of tension and/or have low energy, exercise and improve your eating habits. If, after some time, you don't see the improvement you desire, call a medical practioner for advice and possible testing for low iron, thyroid problems, allergies, stress related illness, or other possible problems. You may also want to talk with a counselor to learn how to deal with internalize pressure.

Faith and spirituality

Spirituality should never 'take a back seat' in the thoughts or concerns of the caregiver, for spirituality is central to the person seeking or requiring our care. The spiritual 'part' is where we live (and die), make decisions, find life's meaning in the midst of those experiences which seem meaningless or to defy meaning or purpose, our sense of values (especially in ethical decision making), and our passageway to that which is eternal for us.
—Rev. Richard B. Gilbert, *A Journey Through Grief: Stepping Stones and Stumbling Blocks*

You may ask yourself, why does this person have to suffer if God is good? You may find it difficult at times to reconcile God's mercy with what may seem like senseless tragedy. You are not alone in this; many caregivers experience this challenge of faith and questioning of God.

If you have a caring faith community, get support from those you believe will understand and help you. If you do not have such a community you may want to ask others to help you find one. If you need guidance and wish to discuss faith issues, talk with a clergyperson. Chances are if you are feeling sad, overwhelmed, depressed or questioning God and the laws of nature, others in your community are also. Maybe by speaking up and sharing your concerns with colleagues, relatives, friends or in support groups, you will find kindred spirits and shared experiences that will empower and touch you.

Read the Bible, the Torah or other spiritual literature. Use prayer, meditation and reflection for comfort. It is understandable to struggle and waiver in your faith, especially when you see people in deep sorrow and pain. You may wonder at God's role in all this and may need to vent your frustration and anger. Struggles are normal, such as wondering why God would allow so much pain and heartache. Remember to also look for God's gifts in all of this. Talk and pray about your feelings and frustrations. Explore and use your faith as a guide in your life. This may be the very foundation on which you gain your strength to go on each day. If it isn't at this time, maybe it could be in the future if you explore this area of your life.

Humor

If you're too busy to laugh, you're entirely too busy.
—Robert Orben

Give yourself permission to laugh and have humor, even in the midst of pain, unless you are so drained of laughter that there is none to be found now. Do use your good judgment about the appropriateness of humor in the presence of those who are hurting. This does not mean it may not have its place, but it is a very sensitive issue that needs careful integration. One can stay serious and intense only for so long. You may need to create opportunities outside of your caregiving for fun and enjoyment.

Smiles and gentle laughter are an antidote to sadness and misery, even if but for a moment. Think about it—often in the midst of a loved one's dying, funny recollections or humorous comments are made at odd moments. Levity provides relief from tension.

It is a fairly accepted belief that laughter is healing, both physically and emotionally. Some say laughter gives your internal organs a massage. When you are feeling especially anxious it may be difficult to have humor, but this is probably one of the most important times to embrace it.

Nurse Mary Funk shares this about humor in her life, "I can't say enough about humor. I consider it one of God's greatest gifts to me. It has gotten me through many difficult situations intact, or so I think—ha! When I've suffered losses, a good chuckle or belly laugh has really eased some of the tension. It doesn't mean I wasn't hurting. Some people act like it is inappropriate to smile amidst the tears, but a laugh provides a breath of fresh air."

Dr. Steve Wilson shares that preschool children laugh over 400 times a day, while many adults laugh on the average only 15 times each day. We need to give ourselves permission to have more humor in our lives. If you can't tell jokes well, read the comics, encourage humor in others and look at your everyday life with an eye for the humorous and absurd. After all, it is all around us. Dr. Wilson suggests that you do not need to "be" funny, but rather "see" funny. Look at yourself and what happens around you in a light manner, seeking the humor to balance the seriousness that is already there.

Relaxation, rest and meditation

Sleep is a vital part of your inner growth. There is a lot going on at the sleep level of consciousness that we are only just beginning to understand. Many spiritual retreat programs include naps, rest time and/or sleep as a major part of the daily regimen. If you've been moving on the fast track in recent years, you may desperately need sleep to restore your body and your mind, not to mention your psyche...So sleep in whenever you can. Go to bed early every night for as long as you need to. Sleep throughout the weekends. Take naps whenever possible. Relish sleep. Luxuriate in it. Grow in it. Expand in it. You need it.
> —Elaine St. James, *Inner Simplicity: 100 Ways to Regain peace and Nourish Your Soul*

Quiet time for contemplation, meditation, prayer and dreams are all important for busy people seeking balance and peace in their lives. Dreams seem to serve a necessary function to our well-being. You must get enough rest in order to have adequate time for dreaming to take place. Dream interpretation is discussed quite a bit these days.

You may find this interesting and stimulating. It's another way to escape your daily duties.

Use relaxation techniques to deal with tight and sore muscles. Learn how to use meditation and make opportunities for quiet times. You may want to check out books and audio/video tapes on the methods of meditation and relaxation from the library or at the bookstore. Find a quiet, distraction-free area, unplug the phone and even dim the lights. Here is an exercise to try:

Play slow, relaxing music, maybe classical, new age or any type that is peaceful, not distracting, to you. Then sit or lie down and beginning at your feet, while breathing in slowly through your nose, tighten your feet, your ankles, calves, thighs, all the way up to your head. Hold tightly (not too tight) then slowly breath out from your mouth and release the pressure and tension from your head, your face, neck, shoulders, arms, fists, etc. all the way down to your toes. Now take deep cleansing breaths. Do this at least three times. Keep in mind that if you feel pain or muscle discomfort keep stop the exercise at any time, or release some of the pressure.

After my mother died there were many nights I could not get to sleep because I was overwhelmed with sad thoughts. To seek calm and rest I would force for my mind to journey to my favorite beach in Hawaii. I felt the sun on my body, heard the waves crashing and invited myself to sink into the sand and relax. Often, though not always, I was able to escape in this way and eventually get to sleep.

Expressing your emotions and seeking calmness

Your worries will vanish if you face them bravely.
                                        —Chinese fortune cookie

What do you do to gain calm, to counter the ills of too much stress, and to recharge your battery? Are you able to face your fears? And how do you express your anger at the unfairness of tragedy, your feelings of inadequacy and frustration, or your own sorrow and pain?

Search for activities that bring you peace, calmness and a chance to escape, even if for but short periods of time. You may want to brainstorm ideas with co-workers, friends and other care providers in your community or at conferences you attend.

Also, ask yourself what advice you give to grieving families—how do you teach them to take care of themselves? What kind of a role model are you? Do you practice what you preach and teach? If you need a little push in getting yourself to the top of your list, you can always say you are doing it for others, so you will be a better caretaker.

✛Create a list of ideas to aid in finding peace in calm in your life. Put them down on paper. ✛ Below are a few suggestions to consider:

- Be as kind to yourself as you are kind to others. You can't help anyone else if you don't take care of yourself first. Do nice things for yourself, you deserve it.
- Exercise, especially walking, is one of the best things you can do. You could also play a team or individual sport.
- Talk with others, your partner, a kindred spirit, a relative, co-worker, or friend.
- Write your feelings in a journal, letters, poetry, or stories.
- Find a closed or safe place and scream, cry, or take many deep breaths.
- Read about ways to help yourself or the people you care for; or read literature that allows you to enter another world and escape
- Play, make or create music. Paint or draw. Use your creativity to express yourself.
- Create something out of wood, clay, or other creative activities.
- Treat yourself to a massage or a hot bath with bubbles, candles and soft music.
- Plan a vacation (the planning can be therapeutic itself), even for a long weekend.
- Go to the theater, movies (you may want to choose a comedy or a subject that is unlike your work), or a dinner out.
- Help someone else, volunteer, or give money to charity.
- Make a list of the things you enjoy doing and be sure that you do them a few times each week.
- Be playful in some way, with your pet, with children, with friends, or by yourself. Find or make an opportunity to be silly and have some fun.
- Do something special for yourself. Put yourself on the calendar

every day. Make *you* a priority!
- Plant a garden. Working in the earth can be therapeutic and relaxing at the time, and again when the flowers or plants bloom and grow.
- Take a walk in the country, near a lake.
- Enjoy a sunset or take note of the sky on a clear night.
- Go shopping for yourself or someone else. Even window shopping can be enjoyable and distracting. You could go sit at a shopping plaza and people watch.
- Do something special with your family. You could take turns letting each one choose what to do.
- Get a pet or if you have one, give your pet some attention. This can be a great stress reliever and some company for you, someone to "talk" with and share your troubles with, someone who is guaranteed not to talk back or try to "fix" you.
- Go dancing or bowling, go to concerts, or even join in on Karoke sessions.
- When you are extremely angry or frustrated, use your breathing to temporarily redirect your thoughts—say the alphabet, count by fours to a thousand, think of pleasant places or favorite books. Channel or expend the anger through pounding clay, or some physical activity.
- Get outside, away from your office and work. A breath of fresh air, a walk in a park, down a country road, or even just on a city street can help you gain a little perspective. There is more to life than just your problem or current experience. Force your mind to take a rest and notice the things around you.
- Escape through a good book, a movie, a play or sporting event.
- Go home and hug your kids, your partner, or another special person.
- Remember something good that you have going for yourself.
- Look in the mirror and give yourself a hug. You deserve it.

Take time to celebrate and appreciate

Have fun celebrating. Find reasons to celebrate and invite others to join in. Celebrate the sunshine, the first snowfall, or any change in the weather for that matter. Celebrate that the office copier didn't jam today! Get the idea? —Steve Wilson, *Super Humor Power*

Celebrate your successes, any and all successes, no matter how small. Also, take notice of and celebrate your progress as well. As a friend's father used to say, "You have got to stop looking at the hole and start looking at the doughnut."

Like most people, you may have times when your lists are so long they run into the next century. There are many reasons to feel overwhelmed—the undone lists, the limited time, the politics at work, living with unresolved losses, the inability to really make someone better, combined with job overload, burnout, or just situational stress. There is so much that can't be done and is not within your power. If you could just "buy more time."

Since we must live with a 24 hour day, of which at least a few hours must be used for sleep, about the only thing we can change is the size of our list and the feelings we have when we do accomplish things, when we make a difference, and when things don't get done right or at all. Most things that really matter weren't on the list anyway—like telling someone we love them, giving a smile of hello or a special thank you to someone.

Take time, make time, to appreciate what you have accomplished, rather than what has been left undone. Whose life have you touched today? Was the sun shining? Did you find a reason to share a smile? Are there things in your life that you can be thankful for? Did you do something today that made a difference? Focus on those things, not what you couldn't or didn't do.

Susan Vineyard suggests at the end of her book, *How to Take Care of You so You Can Take Care of Me*, "There are certain stepping stones that help us on our path toward realizing our fullest potential and greatest health, and we must keep them clearly in sight in our journey through life:"

• Faith in God, a higher power or faith in self and others
• Identification of support from others
• An attitude that is positive and grace-filled
• A zest for living
• An ability to let go
• A realistic assessment of reality
• A list of options
• A healthy sense of humor!
I would like to add:
• Development of many coping skills, including celebrations
   of progress and success
• A helper perspective that encourages heart-to-heart humanness

rather than godlike powers of healing and fixing.

As a caring helper who serves others, you must continually seek balance and good health in an effort to be effective and sensitive. ⊕List three or four things you can celebrate or appreciate. Now take time to celebrate before going on.⊕

When to take a break or seek a new job

Your chances of success are directly proportional to the degree of pleasure you derive from what you do. If you are in a job you hate, face the fact squarely and get out.. —Michael Korda

If you help people in your profession, whether you are paid or volunteer, there will surely come a time when you need a break to recharge your battery or to seek new challenges. Whatever the reasons—burnout, feeling overwhelmed from too much suffering, political or work pressures, a waning interest in the welfare of others, or just exhaustion—when you see the signs pay attention. You may also be getting signals and subtle suggestions from friends, relatives or co-workers. It may be hard to hear these messages. You may resist the idea of a break right now. Financial concerns, self-esteem issues, needing to be needed, and other worries may make it especially difficult take a break, but keep the option open.

Maybe you are living with someone who needs you and you feel you have no other options but to stay at this hard work of caregiving. You do your clients, patients, relatives and yourself no favors when you try to give care but your well is dry, your self-esteem is low, or you have lost the compassion to give them what they need. Seek help from others, take a look at your emotional and physical state and evaluate whether even a short break will help you gain perspective and add energy to your system.

It seems everyone goes through this at some time or another. Maybe all you need is an extended vacation (or lots of long weekends) away from phones, disasters, hard-luck stories and tragedy, where all you have to do is care about yourself and the few people who are with you. Or it may be possible that this job, or this aspect of your job, is no longer right for you. You have changed and grown, you have given and given. Perhaps now is the time to seek other paths that don't involve the continued contact with people in pain. You may find there is a job within your organization or institution or somehow connected to what you do. Or you may need to totally break away.

As a caring relative you may feel your choices are limited. If you don't give this care, who will? This is the question to spend time exploring. Do you have another relative who can share this important job? Could you rotate days, weeks or months? Speak with your clergy, medical care providers or other local resources. Are there volunteers, faith community members or others who can relieve you, even if for hours or a few days at a time? Call a friend to fill in for you for a few hours. Most people are hesitant to ask, yet if you don't people won't know you need help. Consider this a gift to yourself and the person you are caring for. When you return from time away you will probably feel re-energized and have a renewed attitude.

How well are you taking care at this point in your life and where will you go from here? You may use the following evaluation to access your current situation. Then use it to plan for improvement.

Self Care Evaluation

How do you rate?   Check those you do regularly or often:

Physically
___Exercise (walking or more strenuous)
___Eat a well-balanced diet
___Eat low fat and low sodium foods
___Rest when needed
___Sleep at the night
___Other ideas

Emotionally
___Seek help when I need it
___Admit/allow feelings like anger, sadness, guilt and happiness
___Share my feelings with others who can support me
___Seek out a nurturing support network
___Laugh and encourage humor and lightness in my day
___Have and use an outlet for my feelings (e.g. write in journal, sculpting, motorcycle riding, exercise, nature, etc.)
___Handle my personal/family problems and issues in ways that seem appropriate so they don't interfere with my care of others
___Other ways:

Spiritually and giving to others
___Believe in something higher/bigger than myself
___Pray or meditate
___Have and use a faith community to help me when I need it
___Question God, and clergy, expressing feelings
___Practice the "let go, let God" attitude
___Search for ways to give back or make sense of this experience
___Other ways:

Professionally
___Have an understanding regarding the organization's expectations of my professionalism
___Give of myself to others, but have a good balance in my personal/professional life
___Offer my help, but don't try to"rescue"or save"others
___Know and use referral networks and resources
___Ask for support from others when I need it
___Other ways:

What are you good at? Where do you need to grow? Make a commitment to continue the good work in your strong areas and to improve where you have few checks. ✛On paper write a note or a contract as a commitment to put yourself at the top of the priority list. ✛

Remember, you are worth it and this is the greatest gift you can also give others.

Coping advice from other caregivers

Wisdom is acquired through experience and the process of sharing it. The following individuals willingly share their experience in hopes that you might be further inspired.

Michele Prince, M.S.—I have found that as a genetic counselor my life has been dramatically changed by knowing these people who I hope I have helped through the worst time of their lives. The blessing is in the relationship knowing them in a way that many other professionals never get to be a part of. The difficulty is the burden we sometimes feel when we allow ourselves to blow things out of proportion and feel the "weight of the world on our shoulders." When I start to feel like all I ever do is take care of others and listen all day to everyone else's problems, I remind myself that: 1. I am separate—this is not my problem even though I am involved and I care; 2. The rest of the world is still out there—good things do happen even when bad things seem to be everywhere; 3. I look for something good, even if it is a simple hello from a stranger and I do something good, smile at a passerby or help someone find their way; 4. I talk to my friends in genetic counseling and outside of the field—to let go of some of the burden by talking it through.

Gay Summer, New Zealand— "As a counselor of high risk adolescents, a single parent and a university student, I find that my day is full of demands on a number of levels. I have a multi-faceted approach to keeping my life as positive and stress free as possible. It is as follows:

"First, my philosophy of life centers around being positive and always looking for the good in any situation. When I am affected by personal stress I look at what I need to learn from the situation, talk to whomever I need to talk to and then put it behind me. When I am unable to talk I write—whether or not anyone reads it is generally immaterial.

"Second, each day I try to make time to exercise, contemplate and submerge myself in water. I may combine exercise and contemplation by walking or swimming alone. If I go to the gym then I may spend some quiet time in my garden. If I don't swim, I run a deep bath and maybe light a candle or two to relax.

"Walking and gardening help me focus on the beauty of nature. It centers and grounds me, giving me genuine deep pleasure. Water seems to wash away the stress of the day.

"I am very much a goal setter. I write daily, weekly and yearly goals and I love crossing them off. I sometimes write down things I have already done so I can immediately cross them off! I never punish myself for things I did not manage to achieve. Guilt is a feeling I avoid.

"I tend to focus very much on the present—while at work I focus on my client, when at home I focus on my family and our needs.

"I am fortunate to have friends and family who enjoy giving and receiving cuddles and massage. Laughter and touch are the two things I can't do without. I actively seek them out when I realize I have been a bit absent or overwhelmed in my life."

Rev. Richard Gilbert, M.Div., FAAGC, CPBC, Director, Connection-Spiritual Links— "I used think that all of these virtues of love and care were wrapped up in the church. I have seen another side of the church, and it isn't very pretty. I must remind myself of my own shortcomings and above all, that the People of God are bigger than one judicatory leader. But some foolish folks content with power and self-preservation can be very hurtful. It creates voids in the reservoir of love and Love, and increases one's feelings of abandonment or isolation.

"I have been challenged to remind myself of the very definitions of spirituality and religion that I share with others. I remember (and trust) spirituality as connection, as where I find my pathway, my journey, my experience of Love. No one, not even a religious leader, can tamper with that. It is God's gift to me. If religion is above God, then we are all in trouble, and all is meaningless.

41

"The religion will reshape itself, and it will heal. Fortunately, it is community, never one person. The family has risen above it and, one day, I will risk trusting again. It is my wound. The wound will heal.

"All of us, as caregivers, are wounded. We need healing, and we heal not by giving ourselves over to those in our care (though we can share if it is not at the expense of the client), but by our willingness to claim our wounds and tend to them. If we ignore them, they not only fester and grow (just from the magnitude of the stress we are experiencing), but run the risk of hurting others. When we allow room for healing, we grow, and so may those who have come to us for help.

*Barbara Thayer, M.S.—"I have learned over the years that if one is not well and happy, there will be no energy available to give to others, either personally or professionally. I also find that sports like tennis and golf are great stress relievers. I get to take a good whack at something and send it flying. One particular thing I do to give myself a boost is to routinely ask patients to send me baby pictures. It is a real pleasure to get an announcement and I have learned that you get them more often by specifically asking!"

Tim Ryan, husband—I wish I were better at looking out for me but my wife needs me so much. It's a struggle that gets to me sometimes. I cut the grass, play basketball or tennis, remodel something or watch television to get away—anything to occupy my time and redirect my energy.

*Jack Stack, M.D.— "With the death of a spouse, a pastor realizes that the foundation of his belief has been challenged, and he has no pastor to whom he can turn with his doubt and pain. The doctor is not supposed to become ill. The pastor is not to have doubts! The physician or nurse often experience hopelessness and powerlessness when they cannot do enough to fix the problem.

"Professional caregivers use a variety of defenses to deal with intense emotions aroused by our difficult work. We may distance ourselves from our patients or from each other and appear cold and uncaring, or we may make inappropriate and unhealthy attachments with other caregivers or patients. We often use disassociation separating our feelings from our conscious awareness of the intense reality of the situation.

"Another similar defense is intellectualization, which is necessary to practice the science of our professions. We use projection, blaming the patient and each other. We use humor, even joking about disasters in a macabre sort of way as we see on the TV show MASH. To help ourselves we should form professional teams to assist patients and their families. No one professional can do this work alone. We sometimes think we have to, though, and this trap can consume us over time."

*Gail R. Goldberg, RN, MS—"So often our focus as health care professionals is to take care of the patient, not ourselves. When burnout rears its ugly head, we often change jobs or even careers. It is often those aspects that drew us to the profession that cause us to burn out and leave, either emotionally or by changing careers.

"Whenever life's problems get to me, I find solace in my garden. I feel a sense of connectedness to natural cycles. This gives me comfort and centers me. I also get up in the night and watch my son sleep. This renews my hopes for the future."

*Beth Buehler, M.S.—"Every night when I get home I go out for a three mile run. Exercise helps me relieve stress and energizes me after a long day when I am otherwise drained. My husband sometimes accompanies me, but we have a no talking rule during the run. The peace and quiet and rhythm of my footsteps provides the means for my meditation and relaxation. Sometimes I start my run thinking about work, but by the end, my mind is a million miles away as I push my body to make the final sprint home. I find running both exhilarating and medicinal."

Suzanne Helzer, R.N.C., RTS Counselor— "I think we must foster and nurture a strong sense of our own self-worth. If we do not have that sense, then anything we do to take care of ourselves may be accompanied by a sense of guilt, 'Oh, I shouldn't spend that much on myself. I should be getting things done around the house or at work.' The feelings of guilt negate the nurturing we do. So when I play hooky or spend too much time with my nose in a romance novel or buy something that strikes my fancy, I remind myself that I am worth it—and you know what? I am!"

Rhonda Tomai, Counselor—"During the spring and summer months I always begin my day early out in my garden—getting back with nature and connecting to my God. Taking this time before my day starts is most important to me. Getting centered within gives me the capacity to be there with my clients. Also, scheduling time with my family—my parents and sisters—is always a boost for me. Just making the time to visit, eat or play with all the children helps me take a bigger breath of life!"

Catherine Lammert, R.N.,—"Even though I'm a very outgoing person I treasure the peaceful and quiet time of my day. Before I rise in the morning, I take time to meditate and pray."

*excerpts from *Heartbreaking Choice* newsletter, spring 94

In closing...

Many people have shared their thoughts and personal struggles as well as successes. Hopefully you can you relate to some of these people and also be challenged to stretch yourself more in your own growth through caregiving and caretaking.

Though simple concepts—taking and giving good care is far from easy. Each of us must find our own way and determine our priorities in the context of our lives and the changes we go through over time. Believe you can do what you need to do.

You are worth every ounce of effort, so give yourself the gift of care.

Resources

Alzheimer's Association, 919 N. Michigan Ave., Suite 1000, Chicago, IL 60611, (800) 272-3900.

American Cancer Society, 1599 Clifton Road NE, Atlanta, GA30329, (800) ACS-2345.

American Heart Association, 7272 Greenville Ave., Dallas, TX 75231.

American Lung Association, 1740 Broadway, NY, NY 10010, (800) Lung-USA.

American National Red Cross, 17th and D Streets NW, Washington, DC 20006.

American Psychological Association, 750 First Ave. NE, Washington, DC 20002.

A Place to Remember, mail order resources focusing on infant loss for families and care providers. 1885 University Ave., Suite 110, St. Paul, MN 55104, (800) 631-0973.

AARP Widowed Persons Service, 1909 K. St. NW, Washington, DC 20049.

Bereavement Magazine, features articles for and about grief, for all who have dealt with a loss and all who walk with them on that journey. Andrea Gambill, 8133 Telegraph, Colorado Springs, CO 80920.

Canadian Cancer Society, 10 Alcorn Ave., Suite 200, Toronto, Ontario, M4V 3B1.

Canadian Heart Association, 1 Nichols St., Suite 1200, Ottawa, Ontario K1N 7B7.

Canadian Lung Association, 1900 City Park Dr., Suite 508, Blair Business Park, Gloucester, Ontario K1J 1A3.

Canadian Palliative (Hospice) Care Association, 5 Blackburn Ave., Ottawa, Ontario A1N 8A2.

Canadian Psychological Association, 730 Yonge St., Toronto, Ontario M4Y 2BZ.

Canadian Red Cross Society, 1800 Alta Vista Drive, Ottawa, Ontario K1G 4J5

Centering Corporation, newsletter and mail order bookstore with literature on death, dying and coping with bereavement issues, including divorce, illness, disability, death of children, adults and pets. 1531 Saddle Creek Road, Omaha, NE 68104, (402) 553-1200.

Compassion Books/Rainbow Connection, mail order bookstore with resources on grief and related matters. 477 Hannah Branch Road, Burnsville, NC 28714, (704) 675-5909.

Compassionate Friends, Inc., newsletter and chapters for families who have had a child die. PO Box 3696, Oak Brook, IL 60522-3696, (708) 990-0010.

Connections, Dick Gilbert, resources, workshops, and consultation on bereavement, pastoral care, spirituality and health care/ethics. 1504 N. Campbell, Valparaiso, IN 46383, (219) 464-8183.

Grief Letter, a practical newsletter for bereavement caregivers, New England Center for Loss and Transition, PO Box 292, Guilford, CT 06437, (203) 458-1734.

National Hospice Organization, 1901 N. Morre St., Suite 901, Arlington, VA 22209.

RTS Bereavement Services, International perinatal bereavement program, trains professionals and offers support, literature and referrals to support groups and RTS trained health professionals. Gunderson Lutheran Medical Center, 1910 South Ave., LaCrosse, WI 54601, (800) 362-9567, ext. 4747.

Share, Pregnancy and Infant Loss, international organization offers support to care providers and families who experience pregnancy and infant loss, a quarterly newsletter for each group, literature and referrals. St. Joseph's Health Center, 300 First Capitol Dr., St. Charles, MO 63301, (800) 821-6819.

Willowgreen Productions, audio-visual products and literature especially for the caregivers. PO Box 25180, Fort Wayne, IN 46825, (219) 424-7916.

Wintergreen Press, mail order resources, education and referrals on bereavement and infant loss. 3630 Eileen St., Maple Plain, MN 55359, (612) 476-1303.

New Area Code 952

Books and Audio-Visuals

General Wellness, Coping, Caring and Personal Growth

Beattie, Melody, *The Language of Letting Go: Daily Meditations for Codependents*, Hazelden, Harper Collins, 1990.

Burns, Maureen, *Forgiveness: A Gift You Give Yourself*, Empty Enterprises, 1992.

Buscaglia, Leo, *Living, Loving & Learning*, Ballantine Books, 1982.

Carter-Scott, Cherie, *Negaholics: How to Overcome Negativity and Turn Your Life Around*, Fawcett Crest, 1989.

Canfield, Jack and Mark Victor Hansen, *Chicken Soup for the Soul*, Health Communications, Inc., 1993.

Canfield, Jack and Mark Victor Hansen, *A 2nd Helping of Chicken Soup for the Soul*, Health Communications, Inc., 1995.

Cousins Norman, *Anatomy of an Illness*, Bantam Books, 1979.

Dyer, Wayne, *Everyday Wisdom*, Hay House, Inc., 1993.

Ferguson, Bill, *Miracles Are Guaranteed: A Step by Step Guide to Restore Love, Being Free and Creating a Life That Works*, Return to the Heart Publications, PO Box 54183 Houston, TX 77254, 1992.

Finley, Guy, *The Secret of Letting Go*, Llewellyn Publications, 1996.

Floyd, Maita, *CareTakers, The Forgotten People*, Eskualdun Publishers, PO Box 5-266, Phoenix, AZ, 1988.

Gordon, Sol,*When Living Hurts*, Dell, 1988.

Grollman, Earl, *Caring and Coping When Your Loved One is Seriously Ill*, Beacon, 1995.

Helmstetter, Shad, *Choices*, Pocket Books, 1988.

Jaffee, Dennis and Denise Scott, *From Burnout to Balance*, McGraw Hill, 1984.

Jamison, Kaleel, *The Nibble Theory and the Kernel of Power A book about leadership, self-empowerment and personal growth*, Paulest Press, 1984.

Jampolsky, Gerald and Diane Circincione, *Change Your Mind, Change Your Life, Based on a Course in Miracles*, Bantam, 1994.

Jampolsky, Gerald, *Good-Bye to Guilt: Releasing Fear Through Forgiveness*, Bantam, 1995.

Ilardo, Joseph, *Risk-Taking for Personal Growth: A Step by Step Workbook*, New Harbinger Publication, 1992.

Kaufman, Barry Neil, *Happiness is a Choice*, Faucett Columbine, 1991.

Kushner, Rabbi Harold,*When Bad Things Happen to Good People*, Schocken, 1989/91.

Lasher, Margot, *The Art and Practice of Compassion and Empathy*, Tarcher/Putnam, 1992.

Laskars, Leonard, *Healing with Love: A Breakthrough Mind/Body Medical Program for Healing Yourself and Others*, Harper, 1992.

Leider, Richard, *Life Skills Taking Charge of Your Personality and Professional Growth*, Pfeiffer and Company, 1994.

Lerner, Rokelle, *Living in the Comfort Zone, The Gift of Boundaries in Relationships*, Health Communications, 1995.

Littauer, Florence, *Personality Plus: How to Understand Others by Understanding Yourself*, Felming Revell, 1992.

Mallinger, Alan, M.D. and Jeannette DeWyze, *Too Perfect: When Being in Control Gets Out of Control*, Fawcett Columbine, 1992.

Manning, Doug, *Caring for the Caregiver*, audio tape, Insight Books, PO Box 2058, Hereford, TX 79045, (800) 658-9262.

Manning, Doug, *The Quiet Touch: A Course in Caring*, 4 video cassettes:*The Gift of Listening, The Gift of Understanding, The Gift of Comfort, Caring for the Caregiver*, Insight Books.

Maslach, Christina, *Burnout—The Cost of Caring*, Prentice-Hall, 1982.

McCarthy, Kevin, *The On-Purpose Person, Making Your Life Make Sense*, Pinon Press, 1992.

McGinnis, Alan Loy, *The Power of Optimism*, Harper, 1990.

Miller, James E., *How Can I Help, 12 Things to Do When Someone You Know Suffers a Loss*, Willowgreen Productions. PO Box 25180, Fort Wayne, IN 46825.

Moffatt, Betty Claire, *Soulwork: Clearing the Mind, Opening the Heart, Replenishing the Spirit*, Wild Cat Canyon Press, 1994.

Moon, Anna Kaufman and Marion Deutsche Cohen, *Extreme Points: A Collaboration of Words and Images*, Center for Thanatology Research & Education, 391 Atlantic Ave., Brooklyn NY, 11217, 1994.

Moyers, Bill , *Healing & the Mind*, Doubleday, 1993.

Null, Gary, *Be Kind to Yourself Explorations into Self-Empowerment,* Carrol and Graf Publications, 1995.

Peck, M. Scott, *The Road Less Traveled*, Touchstone, 1978.

Peck, M. Scott, *Further Along The Road Less Traveled*, Simon and Schuster, 1993.

Roger, John and Peter McWIlliams, *Life 101: Everything We Wish We Had Learned About Life in School But Didn't*, 1991.

Roger, John, *You Can't Afford the Luxury of a Negative Thought*, Prelude Press, Inc.1991.

Siegel, Bernie S., *Love, Medicine & Miracles: Lessons learned about self-healing from a surgeon's experience with exceptional parents,* Harper & Row, 1986/1990.

Vineyard, Sue, *How to Take Care of You...So You Can Take Care of Others,* Heritage Arts Publishing, 1988.

Weinfeld, Dr. Irwin, *Care for the Caregivers: Coping with Perinatal Death,* Video, Professional Research, 930 Pitner Ave., Evanston, IL 60202.

Williamson, Marianne, *A Return to Love: Reflections on the Principles of A Course in Miracles,* Harper Collins, 1992.

Fitness and Nutrition

Chopra, Deepak, *Perfect Health: The Complete Mind Body Guide,* Harmony Books, 1990.

Douillard, John, Body, *Mind and Sport: The Mind-Body Guide to Lifelong Fitness and Your Personal Best,* Harmony Books, 1994.

Jonas, Steven and Peter Radetsky, *PaceWalking: The Balanced Way to Aerobic Health,* Crown, 1988.

Tubesing, Donald and Nancy Loving Tubesing, *Seeking Your Health Balance,* Whole Person Associates, 1991.

Stress

Greenberg, Jerrold and Wm. C. Brown, *Stress Management,* 1990.

Charlesworth, Edward A. and Ronald G. Nathan, *Stress Management: A Comprehensive Guide to Wellness,* Ballantine Books, 1984.

Davis, Martha, Eshelman and McKay, *The Relaxation and Stress Reduction Workbook,* New Harbinger Publications, 1980.

Gillespie, Peggy Roggenbuck and Lyn Bechtel, *Less Stress in 30 Days: An Integrated Program for Relaxation,* Signet, 1986.

Kirsta, Alix, *The Book of Stess Survival,* Simon and Schuster, 1986.

McKay, Matthew, Davis and Fanning, *The Cognitive Art of Stress Intervention,* New Harbinger Publications, 1981.

Miller, Lyle and Alma Dell Smith, *The Stress Solution,* Pocket, 1993.

Neal, Connie, *52 Ways to Reduce Stress in Your Life,* Thomas Nelson Publications, 1993.

Scott, Dru, *Stress That Motivates,* Crisp Publications, 1992.

Sehnert, Keith W., *Stress/Unstress: How You Can Control Stress at Home and on the Job,* Augsburg, 1981.

Spera, Stefanie and Sandra Lanto, *Beat Stress with Strength: Achieving Wellness at Work and in Life,* DBM Publications.

St. James, Elaine, *Inner Simplicity: 100 Ways to Regain Peace and Nourish Your Soul*, Hyperion, 1995.

Tubesing, Donald A., *Kicking Your Stress Habits: A Do-It-Yourself Guide for Coping With Stress*, Signet, 1981.

Humor

Klein, Allen, *The Healing Power of Humor*, Tarcher-Putnam, 1989.

Wilson, Steve, *Eat Dessert First*, Advocate Publishing Group, 1292 8A, Stonecreek Dr. NW, Pickerington, OH 43147, 1990.

Wilson, Steve, *Super Humor Power*, DPJ Enterprise, Inc. 3400 N. High Street, Suite 120, Columbus, OH 43202.

Sims, Darcie, *Why Are the Casseroles Always Tuna? A Loving Look at the Lighter Side of Grief*, Big A & Company, PO Box 4181, Wenatchee, WA 98807-4181.

Sims, Darcie, *If I Could Just See Hope*, cassette, 1993.

Meditation, relaxation and faith

Cooper, David A., *Silence, Simplicity, and Solitude: A Guide for Spiritual Retreat*, Bell Tower, 1992.

Gawain, Shakti, *Creative Visualization*, Bantam, 1983.

Godwin, Malcolm, *The Lucid Dreamer: A Waking Guide for the Traveller Between Worlds*, Simon & Schuster, 1994.

Goldsmith, Joel, *The Art of Meditation*, Harper, 1956.

Hittleman, Richard, *Guide to Yoga Meditation: The Inner Source of Strength, Security, and Personal Peace*, Bantam, 1969.

Kabot-Zinn, Jon, *Wherever You Go, There You Are: Mindful Meditations in Everyday Life*, Hyperion, 1994.

LaBerge, Stephen, *Lucid Dreaming: The Power of Being Awake & Aware in Your Dreams*, Ballantine, 1985.

Le Shan, Lawrence, *How to Meditate*, Bantam, 1974.

Levine, Stephen, *A Gradual Awakening*, Anchor/Doubleday, 1979.

Lindbergh, Anne Morrow, *Gift from the Sea*, Vintage Books, 1979.

Martinez, Susan Erling, *Angels & Dreams*, Safe & Sound Productions, PO Box 29636, Brooklyn Center, MN 55429.

Ram, Dass, *Journey of Awakening: A Meditator's Guidebook*, Bantam, 1990.

Sadleir, Steven, *The Spiritual Seeker's Guide: The Complete Source for Religions and Spiritual Groups of the World*, Allwon Publishing, 1992.

Silva, Jose with Philip Miele, *The Silva Mind Control Method*, Pocket Books, 1989.

Smith, Jonathan, *Meditation: A Senseless Guide to a Timeless*

Discipline, Research Press, 1986.

Snow, Kimberly, *Keys to the Open Gate: A Woman's Spirituality Sourcebook.* Conari Press, 1994.

Illness, grieving and bereavement

Bozarth-Campbell, Alla, *Life is Goodbye, Life is Hello: Grieving Well Through All Kinds of Losses,* Compcare, 1986.

Buckman, Robert, *How to Break Bad News: A Guide for Health Professionals,* Johns Hopkins University Press, 1992.

Callanan, Maggie and Patrician Kelly, *Final Gifts,* Poseidon Books, 1992.

Cohen, Marion, *The Level of Doorknobs,* Centering Corp., 1994.

Davidson, Glen, *Understanding Mourning,* Augsburg Publishing, 1984.

Grollman, Earl, *Living When a Loved One Has Died,* Beacon.

Hughes, Marylou, *Bereavement and Support: Healing in a Group Environment,* Taylor & Francis, 1995.

Johnson, Elizabeth, *As Someone Dies: A Handbook for the Living,* Hay House, 1985.

Kuenning, Delores, *Helping People Through Grief,* Bethany House Publishers, 1987.

Larson, Dale, *The Helpers Journey: Working with People Facing Grief, Loss and Life-threatening illness,* Research Press, 1993.

Levang, Elizabeth and Sherokee Ilse, *Remembering With Love: Messages of hope for the First Year of Grieving,* Fairview, 1992.

Linn, Erin, *I Know just How You Feel: Avoiding the Cliches of Grief,* The Publisher's Mark, 1986.

Manning, Doug, *Comforting Those Who Grieve,* Insight Books.

Manning, Doug, *Don't Take My Grief Away,* Insight Publications.

Manning, Doug, *Special Care Series, for the first year of grief,* Insight Books.

Pollin, Irene and Susan Golant, *Taking Charge: Overcoming the Challenges of Long Term Illness,* Time, 1994.

Rando, Theresa, *Grieving: How To Go On Living When Someone You Loved Dies,* Heath/Lexington Books, 1988.

Rando, Theresa, *Treatment of Complicated Mourning, Research Press Co.,* 1993.

Simons, Robin, *After the Tears: Talking About Raising a Child with a Disability,* Centering Corporation.

Smith, Joanne and Judy Biggs, *How To Say Goodbye -Working Through Personal Grief,* Aglow Publications, 1990.

Vogel, Gary, *A Caregiver's Handbook to Perinatal Loss,* A Place to Remember, 1996.

Worden, William, *Grief Counseling and Grief Therapy,* Springer Publishing Co., Inc., 1991.

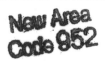